THE CARNIVORE DIET FIX

The Essential Guide to Unlock the Secrets to Maximize Weight Loss and Optimal Health

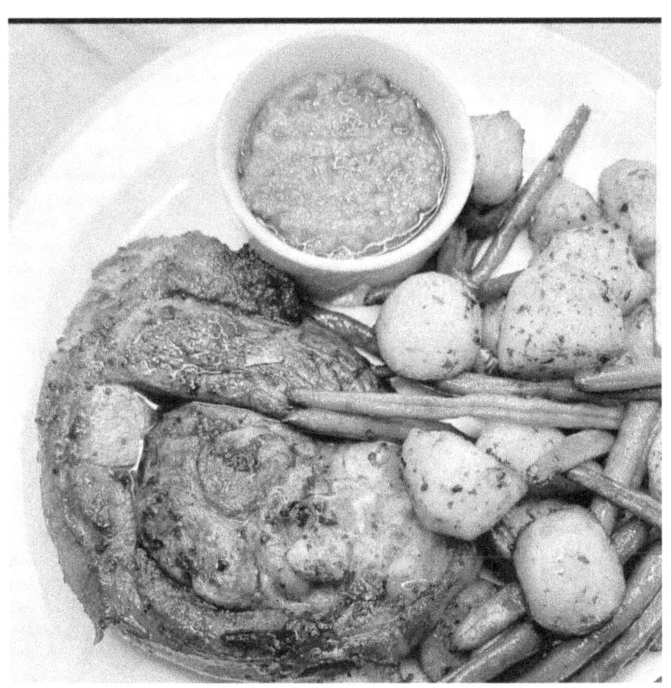

DR. RICHARDSON DAVIDS

TABLE OF CONTENTS

INTRODUCTION

Amidst the multitude of dietary fads and nutritional theories that are out there, the Carnivore Diet stands out as an approachable way to eat that is based on consuming animal products. Welcome to "The Carnivore Diet Fix," a cookbook that goes above the norm and challenges you to go on an amazing culinary adventure that aims to redefine your relationship with food and wellbeing while also tantalizing your taste buds.

We will explore the fundamental ideas of the Carnivore Diet in the pages that follows. This diet promotes the consumption of only animal-based foods, avoiding the intricacies of plant-based nutrition. As we go deeper into the scientific underpinnings and compelling health advantages, "The Carnivore Diet Fix" transforms from a cookbook into a manual for comprehending the tremendous effects that purposeful, animal-centric diet can have on your physical and mental health.

This cookbook is about adopting a lifestyle that connects with our instincts, which forms the basis for good living, rather than about deprivation. Every cuisine in these pages, from tender meat cuts to rich sweets fit for carnivores, is meticulously prepared with a steadfast focus on flavor. Whether you're a devoted follower of the Carnivore Diet for years or a curious outsider, this cookbook is your go-to source for tasty, filling recipes that follow the guidelines of this cutting-edge eating style.

"The Carnivore Diet Fix" is an invitation to experience the fullness of a diet that places an emphasis on nutrient-dense, premium animal products rather than merely a fix. I hope that these dishes become your toolkit for taking back control of your health, encouraging long-lasting vitality, and realizing your potential for a full and active life as we go on this culinary journey together.

Now sharpen your knives, light a fire, and get ready to get obsessed with the craft of carnivorous cooking. Let's set out on a journey where each meal brings us one step closer to living a more vibrant, healthy life—a life where the Carnivore Diet is a source of long-term energy and fulfillment rather than just a temporary solution.

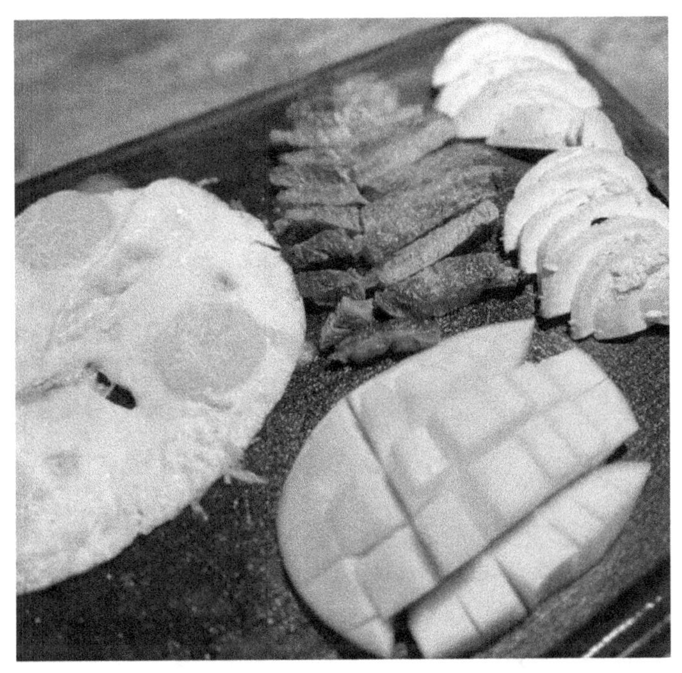

BREAKFAST

BACON AND EGG CUPS

Cooking Time: 15-20 minutes
Nutritional Benefits: High protein, healthy fats.

Ingredients:

Bacon strips

Eggs

Preheat oven to 375°F (190°C).

Line muffin tins with bacon strips.

Crack an egg into each cup.

Bake for 15-20 minutes until eggs are set.

STEAK AND AVOCADO WRAPS

Cooking Time: 10 minutes
Nutritional Benefits: Protein-rich, nutrient-dense.

Ingredients:

Thin steak slices

Avocado slices

Method:

Grill steak slices until cooked.

Wrap steak around avocado slices.

EGG AND SAUSAGE SKILLET

Cooking Time: 15 minutes
Nutritional Benefits: Protein-packed, satiating.

Ingredients:

Eggs

Sausage links

Method:

Brown sausages in a skillet.

Crack eggs into the skillet, cook to desired doneness.

SMOKED SALMON OMELETTE

Cooking Time: 10 minutes
Nutritional Benefits: Omega-3 fatty acids, high-quality protein.

Ingredients:

Eggs

Smoked salmon

Method:

Beat eggs and pour into a hot skillet.

Add smoked salmon, fold, and cook until set.

CHORIZO AND EGG SCRAMBLE

Cooking Time: 15 minutes
Nutritional Benefits: Protein, flavor-packed.

Ingredients:

Chorizo

Eggs

Method:

Cook chorizo in a pan.

Add beaten eggs, scramble until cooked.

KETO COCONUT PANCAKES

Cooking Time: 15 minutes
Nutritional Benefits: Low-carb, high-fiber.

Ingredients:

Coconut flour

Eggs

Method:

Mix coconut flour and eggs into a batter.

Cook small pancakes on a griddle.

CAPRESE BREAKFAST SKILLET

Cooking Time: 10 minutes
Nutritional Benefits: Rich in antioxidants, calcium.

Ingredients:

Cherry tomatoes

Mozzarella

Sauté cherry tomatoes, add mozzarella until melted.

Serve hot.

EGG AND BACON STUFFED AVOCADOS

Cooking Time: 20 minutes
Nutritional Benefits: Healthy fats, protein.

Ingredients:

Avocados

Bacon bits

Method:

Hollow out avocados, stuff with cooked bacon bits and an egg.

Bake until eggs are set.

SARDINE AND EGG SALAD

Cooking Time: 10 minutes
Nutritional Benefits: Omega-3s, protein.

Ingredients:

Canned sardines

Hard-boiled eggs

Method:

Mix flaked sardines and chopped eggs.

Season to taste.

CARNIVORE BREAKFAST BOWL

Cooking Time: 15 minutes
Nutritional Benefits: High-quality protein, satiating.

Ingredients:

Ground beef

Salt and pepper to taste

Cook ground beef in a skillet until browned.

Season and serve.

KETO EGGS BENEDICT

Cooking Time: 15 minutes
Nutritional Benefits: Protein-packed, low-carb.

Ingredients:

Poached eggs

Canadian bacon

Method:

Top Canadian bacon with poached eggs.

Drizzle with hollandaise sauce.

BEEF AND BROCCOLI STIR-FRY

Cooking Time: 10 minutes
Nutritional Benefits: Protein, fiber.

Ingredients:

Thin beef slices

Broccoli florets

Method:

Stir-fry beef and broccoli in a hot pan.

Season to taste.

SPINACH AND BACON EGG MUFFINS

Cooking Time: 15 minutes
Nutritional Benefits: Iron, protein.

Ingredients:

Spinach

Bacon

Method:

Sauté spinach and bacon in a pan.

Pour beaten eggs into muffin cups, add the mixture.

TURKEY AND EGG CUPS

Cooking Time: 20 minutes
Nutritional Benefits: Lean protein, satiating.

Ingredients:

Ground turkey

Eggs

Method:

Mix ground turkey, form into cups in a muffin tin.

Crack an egg into each cup and bake.

LAMB CHOPS WITH ROSEMARY

Cooking Time: 15 minutes
Nutritional Benefits: High-quality protein, aromatic.

Ingredients:

Lamb chops

Fresh rosemary

Method:

Season lamb chops with rosemary, grill to desired doneness.

CAULIFLOWER HASH BROWNS

Cooking Time: 15 minutes
Nutritional Benefits: Low-carb, fiber.

Ingredients:

Grated cauliflower

Eggs

Method:

Mix grated cauliflower and eggs, form into patties.

Cook on a skillet until golden brown.

PORK SAUSAGE PATTIES

Cooking Time: 15 minutes
Nutritional Benefits: Protein, savory.

Ingredients:

Ground pork

Sage and salt to taste

Method:

Mix ground pork with sage and salt, form into patties.

Cook until browned.

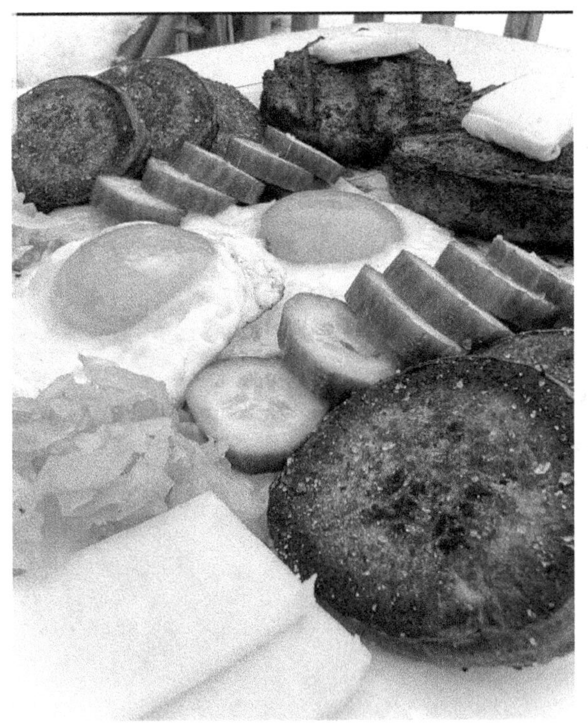

CHICKEN LIVER PÂTÉ

Cooking Time: 15 minutes
Nutritional Benefits: Iron, healthy fats.

Ingredients:

Chicken livers

Butter

Method:

Sauté chicken livers in butter until cooked.

Blend into a smooth pâté.

TURKEY BACON WRAPPED ASPARAGUS

Cooking Time: 20 minutes
Nutritional Benefits: Lean protein, fiber.

Ingredients:

Turkey bacon

Asparagus spears

Method:

Wrap asparagus spears with turkey bacon.

Bake until bacon is crispy.

SALMON AND CREAM CHEESE ROLLS

Cooking Time: 10 minutes
Nutritional Benefits: Omega-3s, high-quality protein.

Ingredients:

Smoked salmon

Cream cheese

Method:

Spread cream cheese on smoked salmon slices.

Roll and secure with toothpicks.

HERB-GRILLED BEEF KEBABS

Cooking Time: 15 minutes
Nutritional Benefits: Protein, aromatic.

Ingredients:

Beef cubes

Fresh herbs (rosemary, thyme)

Skewer beef cubes with fresh herbs.

Grill until desired doneness.

EGG AND CHEESE STUFFED BELL PEPPERS

Cooking Time: 20 minutes
Nutritional Benefits: Protein, vitamins.

Ingredients:

Bell peppers

Eggs

Method:

Hollow out bell peppers, crack an egg into each.

Bake until eggs are set.

SHRIMP AND GARLIC BUTTER

Cooking Time: 10 minutes
Nutritional Benefits: Protein, healthy fats.

Ingredients:

Shrimp

Garlic butter

Method:

Sauté shrimp in garlic butter until pink.

Serve hot.

CRISPY CARNIVORE BURGERS

Cooking Time: 15 minutes
Nutritional Benefits: High-quality protein, satiating.

Ingredients:

Ground beef

Salt and pepper to taste

Form ground beef into patties, season.

Grill until crispy on the outside.

DUCK EGG SALAD WRAPS

Cooking Time: 10 minutes
Nutritional Benefits: Protein, unique flavor.

Ingredients:

Duck eggs

Lettuce leaves

Method:

Hard-boil duck eggs, slice.

Wrap egg slices in lettuce leaves.

TUNA AVOCADO BOATS

Cooking Time: 10 minutes
Nutritional Benefits: Omega-3s, healthy fats.

Ingredients:

Canned tuna

Avocado halves

Method:

Mix tuna with your favorite seasonings.

Fill avocado halves with tuna mixture.

SPICY CHICKEN WINGS

Cooking Time: 30 minutes
Nutritional Benefits: Protein, spicy kick.

Ingredients:

Chicken wings

Hot sauce

Bake or grill chicken wings.

Toss in hot sauce before serving.

HAM AND CHEESE OMELETTE

Cooking Time: 15 minutes
Nutritional Benefits: Protein, calcium.

Ingredients:

Ham slices

Cheese

Method:

Cook ham slices in a pan.

Pour beaten eggs over ham, add cheese, and fold.

SALAMI AND CREAM CHEESE ROLL-UPS

Cooking Time: 10 minutes
Nutritional Benefits: Protein, creamy texture.

Ingredients:

Salami slices

Cream cheese

Method:

Spread cream cheese on salami slices.

Roll and secure with toothpicks.

KETO EGG DROP SOUP

Cooking Time: 10 minutes
Nutritional Benefits: Protein, warming.

Ingredients:

Chicken broth

Eggs

Method:

Heat chicken broth, slowly pour in beaten eggs.

Stir gently until eggs are cooked.

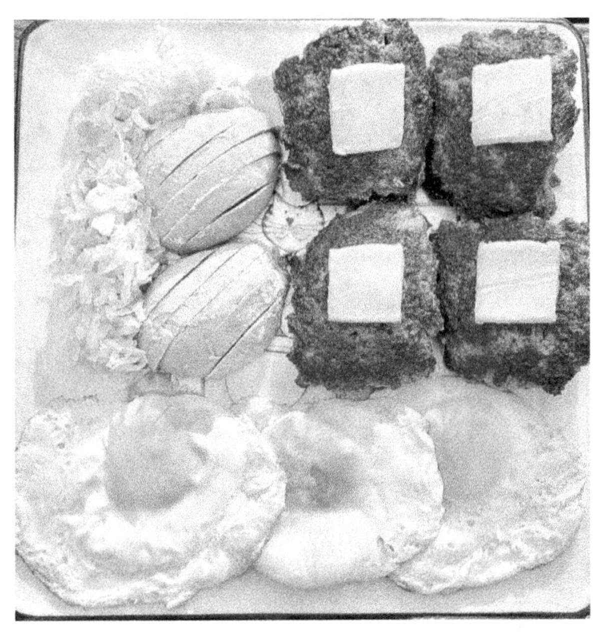

LUNCH

BEEF AND BROCCOLI STIR-FRY

Cooking Time: 10 minutes
Nutritional Benefits: High-quality protein, fiber.

Ingredients:

Thin beef slices

Broccoli florets

Method:

Stir-fry beef and broccoli in a hot pan.

Season to taste.

CHICKEN CAESAR SALAD

Cooking Time: 15 minutes
Nutritional Benefits: Protein, vitamins.

Ingredients:

Grilled chicken breast

Romaine lettuce

Method:

Toss grilled chicken over chopped romaine.

Dress with Caesar dressing.

EGG DROP SOUP WITH CHICKEN

Cooking Time: 10 minutes
Nutritional Benefits: Protein, warming.

Ingredients:

Chicken broth

Eggs

Method:

Heat chicken broth, slowly pour in beaten eggs.

Stir gently until eggs are cooked.

GRILLED SALMON WITH LEMON

Cooking Time: 15 minutes
Nutritional Benefits: Omega-3s, high-quality protein.

Ingredients:

Salmon fillets

Lemon slices

Grill salmon with lemon slices until cooked.

Season to taste.

TURKEY AVOCADO LETTUCE WRAPS

Cooking Time: 10 minutes
Nutritional Benefits: Lean protein, healthy fats.

Ingredients:

Sliced turkey breast

Avocado slices

Method:

Wrap turkey slices around avocado.

Secure with toothpicks.

SHRIMP AND AVOCADO SALAD

Cooking Time: 10 minutes
Nutritional Benefits: Protein, healthy fats.

Ingredients:

Shrimp

Avocado cubes

Method:

Sauté shrimp, toss with avocado cubes.

Season to taste.

BACON-WRAPPED CHICKEN THIGHS

Cooking Time: 25 minutes
Nutritional Benefits: Protein, savory.

Ingredients:

Chicken thighs

Bacon strips

Wrap bacon around chicken thighs.

Bake until both are cooked.

LAMB SALAD WITH MINT DRESSING

Cooking Time: 15 minutes
Nutritional Benefits: Protein, refreshing.

Ingredients:

Grilled lamb chops

Mixed greens

Method:

Arrange mixed greens, top with grilled lamb chops.

Drizzle with mint dressing.

TUNA STUFFED AVOCADO HALVES

Cooking Time: 10 minutes
Nutritional Benefits: Omega-3s, high-quality protein.

Ingredients:

Canned tuna

Avocado halves

Method:

Mix tuna with your favorite seasonings.

Fill avocado halves with tuna mixture.

SPICY SAUSAGE STIR-FRY

Cooking Time: 15 minutes
Nutritional Benefits: Protein, bold flavors.

Ingredients:

Spicy sausage

Bell peppers

Method:

Sauté spicy sausage and bell peppers.

Season to taste.

CAULIFLOWER RICE WITH GROUND BEEF

Cooking Time: 15 minutes
Nutritional Benefits: Protein, low-carb.

Ingredients:

Ground beef

Cauliflower rice

Method:

Cook ground beef, mix with cauliflower rice.

Season to taste.

EGGPLANT LASAGNA

Cooking Time: 30 minutes
Nutritional Benefits: Protein, low-carb.

Ingredients:

Ground beef

Sliced eggplant

Method:

Layer sliced eggplant with cooked ground beef.

Bake until eggplant is tender.

CHICKEN ZOODLE STIR-FRY

Cooking Time: 15 minutes
Nutritional Benefits: Protein, low-carb.

Ingredients:

Zucchini noodles (zoodles)

Grilled chicken strips

Method:

Sauté zoodles with grilled chicken.

Season to taste.

PORK CHOP SALAD

Cooking Time: 20 minutes
Nutritional Benefits: Protein, vitamins.

Ingredients:

Grilled pork chops

Mixed greens

Method:

Arrange mixed greens, top with grilled pork chops.

Dress with vinaigrette.

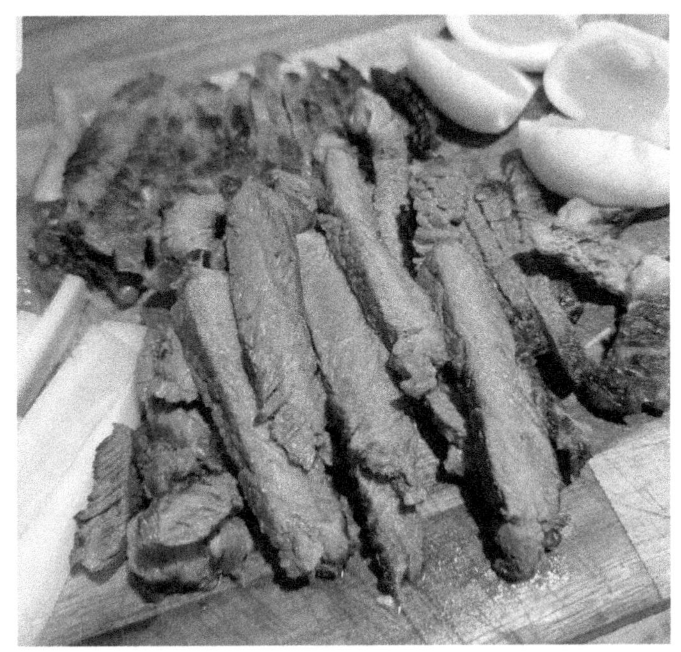

TURKEY BROCCOLI CASSEROLE

Cooking Time: 25 minutes
Nutritional Benefits: Protein, fiber.

Ingredients:

Ground turkey

Broccoli florets

Method:

Cook ground turkey, mix with steamed broccoli.

Bake until golden brown.

SALAMI AND CHEESE PLATE

Cooking Time: 5 minutes
Nutritional Benefits: Protein, satiating.

Ingredients:

Assorted salami slices

Cheese cubes

Method:

Arrange salami and cheese on a plate.

Serve as a quick and satisfying lunch.

EGG SALAD LETTUCE WRAPS

Cooking Time: 10 minutes
Nutritional Benefits: Protein, low-carb.

Ingredients:

Hard-boiled eggs

Lettuce leaves

Chop eggs, mix with your favorite seasonings.

Wrap egg salad in lettuce leaves.

GRILLED CHICKEN KEBABS

Cooking Time: 15 minutes
Nutritional Benefits: Protein, vitamins.

Ingredients:

Chicken breast cubes

Bell peppers

Method:

Skewer chicken cubes with bell peppers.

Grill until chicken is cooked through.

TUNA AND OLIVE SALAD

Cooking Time: 10 minutes
Nutritional   Benefits: Omega-3s,
savory.

Ingredients:

Canned tuna

Sliced olives

Method:

Mix tuna with sliced olives.

Season to taste.

BACON-WRAPPED ASPARAGUS

Cooking Time: 20 minutes
Nutritional Benefits: Fiber, savory.

Ingredients:

Asparagus spears

Bacon strips

Method:

Wrap asparagus with bacon.

Bake until bacon is crispy.

SARDINE SALAD WITH AVOCADO

Cooking Time: 10 minutes
Nutritional Benefits: Omega-3s, healthy fats.

Ingredients:

Canned sardines

Avocado cubes

Method:

Mix flaked sardines with avocado cubes.

Season to taste.

CABBAGE AND SAUSAGE STIR-FRY

Cooking Time: 15 minutes
Nutritional Benefits: Fiber, protein.

Ingredients:

Cabbage

Sausage links

Method:

Sauté cabbage and sausage in a pan.

Season to taste.

STEAK SALAD WITH BLUE CHEESE DRESSING

Cooking Time: 15 minutes
Nutritional Benefits: Protein, calcium.

Ingredients:

Grilled steak slices

Mixed greens

Arrange mixed greens, top with grilled steak slices.

Drizzle with blue cheese dressing.

CARNIVORE AVOCADO BOATS

Cooking Time: 15 minutes
Nutritional Benefits: Protein, healthy fats.

Ingredients:

Ground beef

Avocado halves

Method:

Cook ground beef, fill avocado halves.

Season to taste.

BUTTERY LEMON GARLIC SHRIMP

Cooking Time: 10 minutes
Nutritional Benefits: Protein, flavor-packed.

Ingredients:

Shrimp

Butter, lemon, garlic

Method:

Sauté shrimp in butter, lemon, and garlic.

Season to taste.

PORK RIND CRUSTED CHICKEN NUGGETS

Cooking Time: 20 minutes
Nutritional Benefits: Protein, crunchy texture.

Ingredients:

Chicken breast nuggets

Crushed pork rinds

Coat chicken nuggets in crushed pork rinds.

Bake until crispy.

LIVER AND ONIONS

Cooking Time: 15 minutes
Nutritional Benefits: Iron, protein.

Ingredients:

Beef liver

Sliced onions

Method:

Sauté beef liver and onions until cooked.

Season to taste.

SPINACH AND BACON SALAD

Cooking Time: 10 minutes
Nutritional Benefits: Iron, savory.

Ingredients:

Spinach leaves

Bacon bits

Method:

Toss spinach with bacon bits.

Dress with your favorite vinaigrette.

TURKEY BACON AND EGG MUFFINS

Cooking Time: 15 minutes
Nutritional Benefits: Protein, low-carb.

Ingredients:

Turkey bacon

Eggs

Method:

Line muffin tins with turkey bacon.

Crack an egg into each cup and bake.

CARNIVORE CAULIFLOWER CASSEROLE

Cooking Time: 25 minutes
Nutritional Benefits: Protein, low-carb.

Ingredients:

Ground beef

Cauliflower florets

Method:

Cook ground beef, mix with steamed cauliflower.

Bake until golden brown.

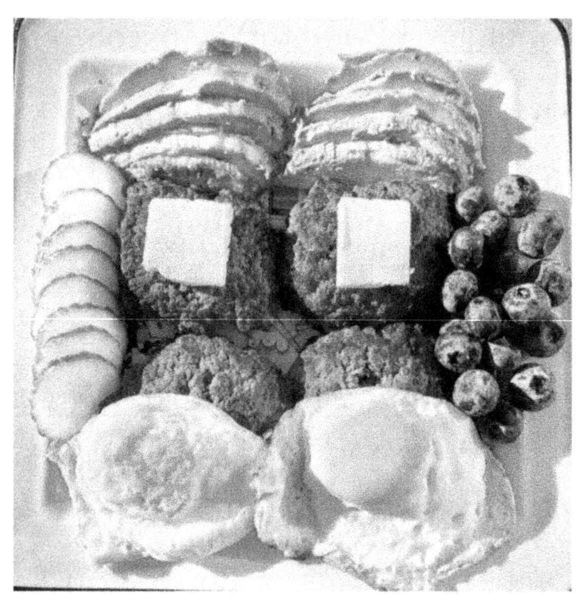

DINNER

GRILLED RIBEYE STEAK

Cooking Time: 15 minutes
Nutritional Benefits: High-quality protein, iron.

Ingredients:

Ribeye steak

Salt and pepper to taste

Season ribeye with salt and pepper.

Grill to desired doneness.

SALMON AND ASPARAGUS BAKE

Cooking Time: 20 minutes
Nutritional Benefits: Omega-3s, fiber.

Ingredients:

Salmon fillets

Asparagus spears

Method:

Place salmon and asparagus on a baking sheet.

Bake until salmon is cooked through.

CAULIFLOWER MASHED "POTATOES"

Cooking Time: 15 minutes
Nutritional Benefits: Low-carb, fiber.

Ingredients:

Cauliflower

Butter

Method:

Steam cauliflower, mash with butter.

Season to taste.

BEEF BURGER SALAD

Cooking Time: 15 minutes
Nutritional Benefits: Protein, vitamins.

Ingredients:

Ground beef

Mixed salad greens

Grill beef patties, serve over salad greens.

Dress with your favorite vinaigrette.

PORK CHOP WITH ROSEMARY BUTTER

Cooking Time: 25 minutes
Nutritional Benefits: Protein, aromatic.

Ingredients:

Pork chops

Fresh rosemary

Method:

Sear pork chops with fresh rosemary.

Finish in the oven until cooked.

TURKEY STUFFED BELL PEPPERS

Cooking Time: 30 minutes
Nutritional Benefits: Lean protein, vitamins.

Ingredients:

Ground turkey

Bell peppers

Method:

Cook ground turkey, stuff into bell peppers.

Bake until peppers are tender.

SHRIMP SCAMPI

Cooking Time: 10 minutes
Nutritional Benefits: Protein, healthy fats.

Ingredients:

Shrimp

Garlic butter

Method:

Sauté shrimp in garlic butter until pink.

Season to taste.

EGGPLANT LASAGNA

Cooking Time: 30 minutes
Nutritional Benefits: Protein, low-carb.

Ingredients:

Ground beef

Sliced eggplant

Layer sliced eggplant with cooked ground beef.

Bake until eggplant is tender.

DUCK BREAST WITH BERRY GLAZE

Cooking Time: 20 minutes
Nutritional Benefits: Protein, antioxidants.

Ingredients:

Duck breast

Mixed berries

Method:

Sear duck breast, make a berry glaze.

Serve with the glaze.

CARNIVORE STIR-FRY

Cooking Time: 15 minutes
Nutritional **Benefits:** High-quality protein, fiber.

Ingredients:

Beef strips

Broccoli florets

Method:

Sauté beef strips and broccoli in a hot pan.

Season to taste.

CABBAGE AND BACON STIR-FRY

Cooking Time: 15 minutes
Nutritional Benefits: Fiber, savory.

Ingredients:

Cabbage

Bacon bits

Sauté cabbage and bacon in a pan.

Season to taste.

SALMON AVOCADO BOATS

Cooking Time: 20 minutes
Nutritional Benefits: Omega-3s, healthy fats.

Ingredients:

Salmon fillets

Avocado halves

Method:

Grill salmon, fill avocado halves.

Season to taste.

CHICKEN THIGH SKILLET

Cooking Time: 25 minutes
Nutritional Benefits: Protein, rich flavor.

Ingredients:

Chicken thighs

Salt and pepper to taste

Method:

Sear chicken thighs in a skillet.

Finish in the oven until cooked through.

TUNA STEAKS WITH LEMON GARLIC BUTTER

Cooking Time: 15 minutes
Nutritional Benefits: Protein, flavor-packed.

Ingredients:

Tuna steaks

Lemon garlic butter

Sear tuna steaks, drizzle with lemon garlic butter.

Cook to desired doneness.

SPICY SAUSAGE STUFFED MUSHROOMS

Cooking Time: 20 minutes
Nutritional Benefits: Protein, bold flavors.

Ingredients:

Spicy sausage

Mushrooms

Method:

Cook spicy sausage, stuff into mushrooms.

Bake until mushrooms are tender.

BEEF LIVER PÂTÉ

Cooking Time: 15 minutes
Nutritional Benefits: Iron, healthy fats.

Ingredients:

Beef liver

Butter

Method:

Sauté beef liver in butter until cooked.

Blend into a smooth pâté.

CRISPY CHICKEN THIGHS WITH SPINACH

Cooking Time: 25 minutes
Nutritional Benefits: Protein, iron.

Ingredients:

Chicken thighs

Fresh spinach

Method:

Roast chicken thighs until crispy.

Serve over sautéed spinach.

BACON-WRAPPED CHICKEN BREAST

Cooking Time: 25 minutes
Nutritional Benefits: Protein, savory.

Ingredients:

Chicken breast

Bacon strips

Method:

Wrap chicken breast with bacon.

Bake until chicken is cooked through.

KETO BEEF AND BROCCOLI

Cooking Time: 15 minutes
Nutritional Benefits: High-quality protein, fiber.

Ingredients:

Thin beef slices

Broccoli florets

Method:

Stir-fry beef and broccoli in a hot pan.

Season to taste.

SALAMI AND CHEESE STUFFED BELL PEPPERS

Cooking Time: 20 minutes
Nutritional Benefits: Protein, calcium.

Ingredients:

Salami slices

Cheese

Cut bell peppers in half, stuff with salami and cheese.

Bake until peppers are tender.

CARNIVORE MEATBALLS

Cooking Time: 20 minutes
Nutritional Benefits: Protein, satiating.

Ingredients:

Ground beef

Salt and pepper to taste

Method:

Form ground beef into meatballs, season.

Bake until browned and cooked through.

TURKEY BACON-WRAPPED ASPARAGUS BUNDLES

Cooking Time: 20 minutes
Nutritional Benefits: Lean protein, fiber.

Ingredients:

Turkey bacon

Asparagus spears

Method:

Wrap asparagus with turkey bacon.

Bake until bacon is crispy.

CARNIVORE STUFFED MUSHROOM CAPS

Cooking Time: 20 minutes
Nutritional Benefits: Protein, savory.

Ingredients:

Ground beef

Mushrooms caps

Cook ground beef, stuff into mushroom caps.

Bake until mushrooms are tender.

LAMB KABOBS WITH MINT YOGURT SAUCE

Cooking Time: 15 minutes
Nutritional Benefits: Protein, refreshing.

Lamb cubes

Fresh mint

Skewer lamb cubes with fresh mint.

Grill until desired doneness.

CARNIVORE BEEF CABBAGE ROLLS

Cooking Time: 30 minutes
Nutritional Benefits: Protein, low-carb.

Ingredients:

Ground beef

Cabbage leaves

Method:

Cook ground beef, wrap in cabbage leaves.

Bake until cabbage is tender.

EGG DROP SOUP WITH BEEF

Cooking Time: 10 minutes
Nutritional Benefits: Protein, warming.

Ingredients:

Beef broth

Eggs

Heat beef broth, slowly pour in beaten eggs.

Stir gently until eggs are cooked.

SARDINE AND AVOCADO SALAD

Cooking Time: 10 minutes
Nutritional Benefits: Omega-3s, healthy fats.

Ingredients:

Canned sardines

Avocado cubes

Method:

Mix flaked sardines with avocado cubes.

Season to taste.

CARNIVORE CABBAGE STIR-FRY

Cooking Time: 15 minutes
Nutritional Benefits: Protein, fiber.

Ingredients:

Ground beef

Shredded cabbage

Method:

Sauté ground beef and cabbage in a pan.

Season to taste.

CHICKEN LIVER AND ONIONS

Cooking Time: 15 minutes
Nutritional Benefits: Iron, protein.

Ingredients:

Chicken livers

Sliced onions

Method:

Sauté chicken livers and onions until cooked.

Season to taste.

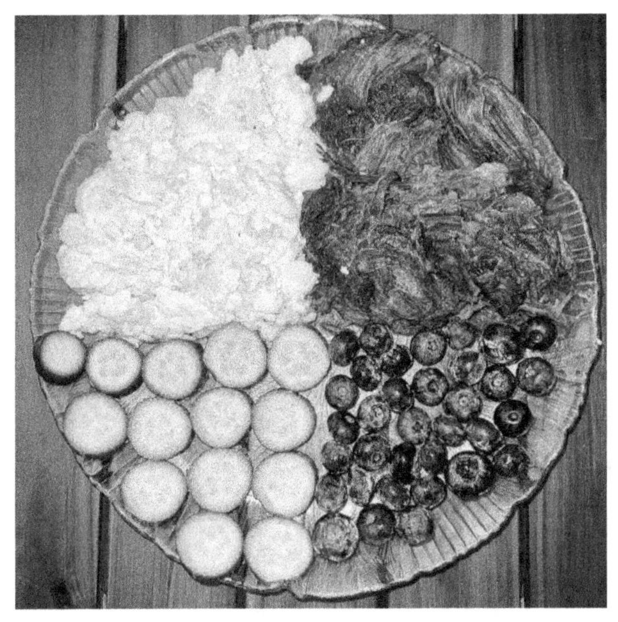

SNACKS

BACON-WRAPPED AVOCADO BITES

Cooking Time: 15 minutes
Nutritional Benefits: Healthy fats, savory.

Ingredients:

Avocado slices

Bacon strips

Method:

Wrap each avocado slice with a bacon strip.

Bake until bacon is crispy.

CARNIVORE CHEESE CRISPS

Cooking Time: 10 minutes
Nutritional Benefits: Calcium, crunchy texture.

Ingredients:

Cheese slices

Method:

Place cheese slices on a parchment-lined tray.

Bake until edges are golden brown.

PEPPERONI AND CREAM CHEESE ROLL-UPS

Cooking Time: 5 minutes
Nutritional Benefits: Protein, creamy texture.

Ingredients:

Pepperoni slices

Cream cheese

Method:

Spread cream cheese on pepperoni slices.

Roll and secure with toothpicks.

CARNIVORE EGG SALAD

Cooking Time: 10 minutes
Nutritional Benefits: Protein, satiating.

Ingredients:

Hard-boiled eggs

Mayonnaise

Chop hard-boiled eggs, mix with mayonnaise.

Season to taste.

BEEF JERKY

Cooking Time: 4-6 hours (dehydrating)
Nutritional Benefits: High-quality protein, portable.

Ingredients:

Beef slices

Salt and pepper to taste

Method:

Marinate beef slices in salt and pepper.

Dehydrate until jerky consistency is achieved.

CARNIVORE CAPRESE SKEWERS

Cooking Time: 10 minutes
Nutritional Benefits: Protein, fresh flavors.

Ingredients:

Cherry tomatoes

Mozzarella balls

Basil leaves

Method:

Skewer tomatoes, mozzarella, and basil.

Drizzle with olive oil.

SARDINE STUFFED CUCUMBER ROUNDS

Cooking Time: 5 minutes
Nutritional Benefits: Omega-3s, refreshing.

Ingredients:

Cucumber rounds

Canned sardines

Method:

Place sardines on cucumber rounds.

Season to taste.

CAULIFLOWER HUMMUS WITH PORK RINDS

Cooking Time: 15 minutes
Nutritional Benefits: Low-carb, satisfying.

Ingredients:

Cauliflower

Olive oil

Pork rinds

Method:

Blend cauliflower with olive oil until smooth.

Serve with pork rinds.

CARNIVORE CHEESEBURGER BITES

Cooking Time: 10 minutes
Nutritional Benefits: Protein, flavorful.

Ingredients:

Ground beef

Cheese cubes

Method:

Form small beef patties, place a cube of cheese in the center.

Cook until beef is browned and cheese is melted.

CHICKEN AVOCADO LETTUCE WRAPS

> **Cooking Time:** 10 minutes
> **Nutritional Benefits:** Protein, healthy fats.

Ingredients:

Rotisserie chicken, shredded

Avocado slices

Lettuce leaves

Method:

Place shredded chicken and avocado on lettuce leaves.

Wrap and secure with toothpicks.

MEAL PLAN

Day 1:

- **Breakfast:** Scrambled Eggs with Bacon
- **Lunch:** Grilled Chicken Caesar Salad
- **Dinner:** Ribeye Steak with Buttered Asparagus

Day 2:

- **Breakfast:** Carnivore Cheese Crisps
- **Lunch:** Tuna Avocado Boats
- **Dinner:** Lamb Chops with Rosemary Butter

Day 3:

- **Breakfast:** Carnivore Egg Salad
- **Lunch:** Beef and Broccoli Stir-Fry
- **Dinner:** Salmon and Creamy Cabbage

Day 4:

- **Breakfast:** Sardine and Avocado Salad

- **Lunch:** Turkey Bacon-Wrapped Asparagus Bundles

- **Dinner:** Pork Rind Crusted Chicken Nuggets

Day 5:

- **Breakfast:** Bacon-Wrapped Avocado Bites

- **Lunch:** Carnivore Cheeseburger Bites

- **Dinner:** Grilled Salmon with Lemon and Spinach

Day 6:

- **Breakfast:** Carnivore Caprese Skewers

- **Lunch:** Chicken Liver Pâté with Cucumber Slices

- **Dinner:** Beef Liver and Onions

Day 7:

- **Breakfast:** Egg Drop Soup with Beef

- **Lunch:** Carnivore Stuffed Mushroom Caps

- **Dinner:** Chicken Thigh Skillet with Broccoli

Day 8:

- **Breakfast:** Beef Jerky

- **Lunch:** Turkey Stuffed Bell Peppers

- **Dinner:** Tuna Steaks with Lemon Garlic Butter

Day 9:

- **Breakfast:** Carnivore Hummus with Pork Rinds

- **Lunch:** Spicy Sausage Stuffed Mushrooms

- **Dinner:** Grilled Chicken Kebabs with Mixed Greens

Day 10:

- **Breakfast:** Carnivore Cheese Crisps

- **Lunch:** Shrimp Scampi with Zucchini Noodles

- **Dinner:** Beef and Broccoli Stir-Fry

Day 11:

- **Breakfast:** Bacon-Wrapped Avocado Bites

- **Lunch:** Carnivore Meatballs with Tomato Sauce

- **Dinner:** Salmon and Asparagus Bake

Day 12:

- **Breakfast:** Egg Salad Lettuce Wraps

- **Lunch:** Pork Chop Salad

- **Dinner:** Chicken Liver and Onions

Day 13:

- **Breakfast:** Sardine Stuffed Cucumber Rounds

- **Lunch:** Carnivore Cabbage Stir-Fry

- **Dinner:** Tuna and Olive Salad

Day 14:

- **Breakfast:** Carnivore Cheeseburger Bites

- **Lunch:** Turkey Bacon and Egg Muffins

- **Dinner:** Ribeye Steak with Buttered Asparagus

Day 15:

- **Breakfast:** Carnivore Cheese Crisps

- **Lunch:** Grilled Chicken Caesar Salad

- **Dinner:** Lamb Chops with Rosemary Butter

Day 16:

- **Breakfast:** Carnivore Egg Salad

- **Lunch:** Beef and Broccoli Stir-Fry

- **Dinner:** Salmon and Creamy Cabbage

Day 17:

- **Breakfast:** Sardine and Avocado Salad

- **Lunch:** Turkey Bacon-Wrapped Asparagus Bundles

- **Dinner:** Pork Rind Crusted Chicken Nuggets

Day 18:

- **Breakfast:** Bacon-Wrapped Avocado Bites

- **Lunch:** Carnivore Cheeseburger Bites

- **Dinner:** Grilled Salmon with Lemon and Spinach

Day 19:

- **Breakfast:** Carnivore Caprese Skewers

- **Lunch:** Chicken Liver Pâté with Cucumber Slices

- **Dinner:** Beef Liver and Onions

Day 20:

- **Breakfast:** Egg Drop Soup with Beef

- **Lunch:** Carnivore Stuffed Mushroom Caps

- **Dinner:** Chicken Thigh Skillet with Broccoli

Day 21:

- **Breakfast:** Beef Jerky

- **Lunch:** Turkey Stuffed Bell Peppers

- **Dinner:** Tuna Steaks with Lemon Garlic Butter

Note: Adjust portion sizes according to your individual nutritional needs and consult with a healthcare professional before starting any new diet plan. Additionally, ensure adequate hydration and consider supplementing with electrolytes if needed.

CONCLUSION

You should be proud of yourself for making the commitment to your health and wellbeing that is a carnivorous diet. As you come to the end of this life-changing event, pause to consider how committed you have been to learning about a distinct and methodical approach to eating. Every meal was a step toward a deeper understanding of what your body needed, whether you embraced the rich flavors of succulent meats, savored in the simplicity of cheese crackers, or enjoyed the freshness of seafood.

I hope that the knowledge you gained from this carnivorous experience will help you in your continued pursuit of a healthy, well-rounded lifestyle. Keep in mind that maintaining your health is a dynamic process, and the vitality you experience today is influenced by the decisions you make today. May you continue to learn, make thoughtful decisions, and achieve the overall well-being you want to in the future.

I hope your road ahead is filled with vigor, strength, and long-lasting health. I'm toasting to your health and wishing you many years of happiness and prosperity.

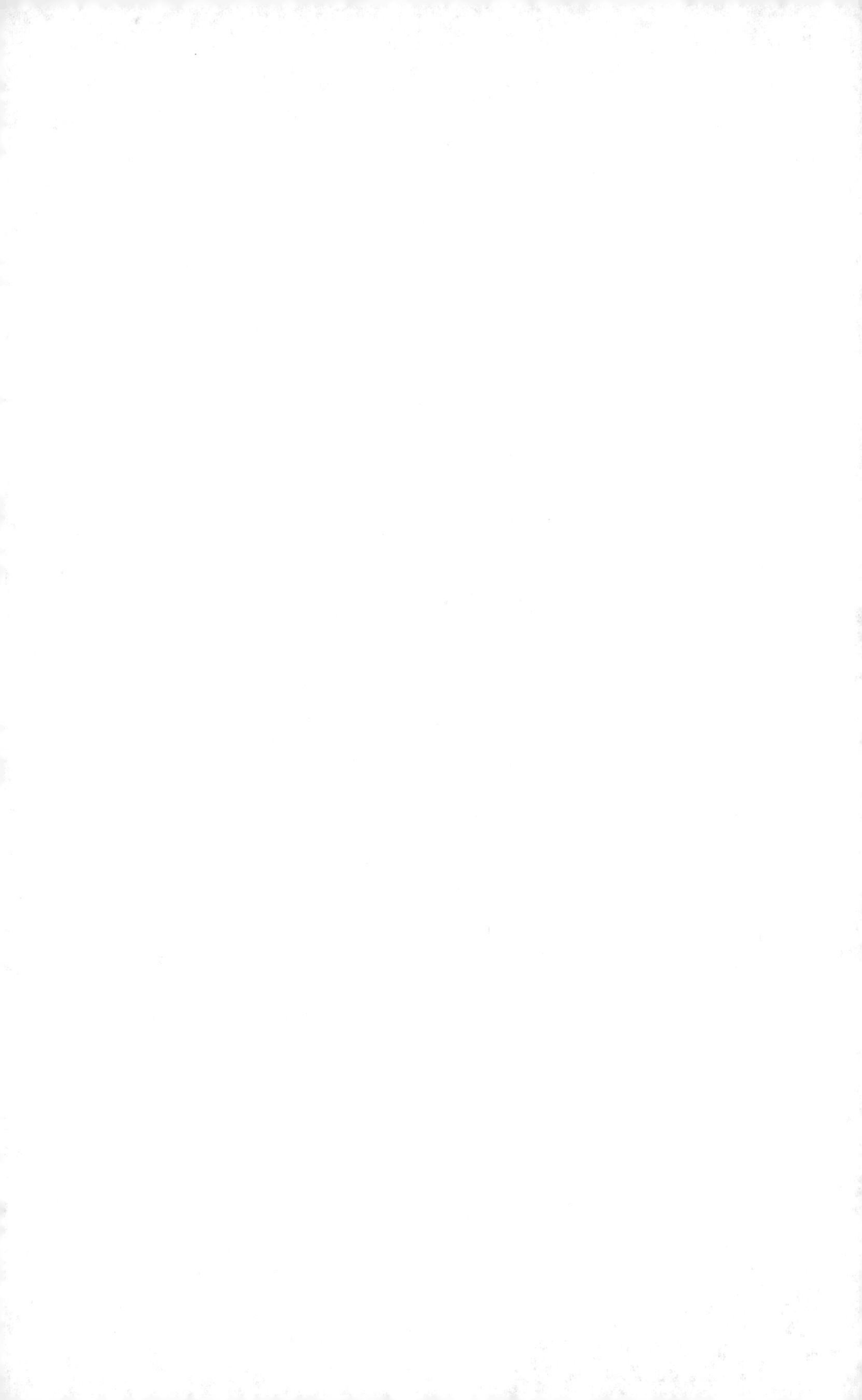